Juicing:
The Ultimate Beginners Guide
for Juicing With the Ninja
& Nutribullet

Easy to Follow Juicing Recipes
for Rapid Weight Loss, Fat Loss,
High Energy, Great Skin, and
a Lean-Fit Body.

Sione Michelson

Disclaimer

Check Out My Other Books

Paleo Diet: 7 Days To Better Health: Cure Your Acid Reflux, Heartburn, Start losing Weight, Lower Blood Pressure and Cholesterol All in a Week through ... Diet, Slow Cooker, Recipes, Diet Recipes)

Paleo Diet: Why The Paleo Diet is better for you than the Low Fat High Carb Diet & the Paleo Recipes that will help Save Your Life! (Paleo Cookbook, Weight-Loss, ... Diet, Slow Cooker, Recipes, Diet Recipes)

Paleo Diet: Learn How to Lose Weight and Feel Amazing in just 5 Short Weeks.The Quickest way to Fit into that Swimsuit for Summer! (Paleo Made Easy) (Paleo ... Diet, Slow Cooker, Recipes, Diet Recipes)

Highlights!

12. Six Pack, No More Keg

- 1/2 avocado
- 1 green apple
- 1 cup spinach
- 1 handful parsley
- 1/2 cup of kale
- 1/2 cup blue berries

Health Benefit:

Studies have shown that consuming blueberries helps individuals maintain optimal health because they contain vital nutrients the body desperately needs especially since the diets of most Americans today consist of mostly processed foods. Blue berries help improve memory, boost the immune system, improve eye sight and **neutralize free radicals.** These tasty little treats are packed with *Anthocyanin* which is found in the dark blue color of the blueberries. This powerful antioxidant helps neutralize free radicals that can lead to cancer and other diseases.

16. Curves in All the Right Places

- — 1 avocado
- — 1 handful of mint
- — 1 cup spinach
- — 1 cup parsley
- — 1/2 cup of strawberries

Health Benefit: Avocados are high in beta-sitosterol, a compound that has been shown to lower cholesterol levels. I love to add avocados to most of my juices because they are a great source of protein which is great for muscle recovery after an intense workout.

Table of Contents

---

1. Introduction

First of all I want to thank you for purchasing my book but you should really be thanking yourself for taking the initiative towards good health. I know your body will be thanking you when your blood pressure is back to normal and your bad cholesterol is out of the danger zone because you decided to take in all the health benefits from juicing. The fat cells in your body may be cussing you out as they die an agonizing death but that's kind of the point right? It's time to get back to nature and consume the right foods that the body utilizes to naturally shed excess weight and bring you back to optimal health.

My own personal experiences with juicing have been phenomenal. Consuming these juices from these recipes along with other minor lifestyle changes has helped me shed the extra weight very easily. I only consumed protein and juiced with fruits and veggies and the weight just fell off. To be perfectly honest, I hardly ever exercised. It's almost like I gave my body exactly what it needed to turn on my fat burning engine and once it started it just keep going!

I'm not promising that these juices will instantly help you lose weight or cure a disease but there is no question that it surely won't hurt your progression towards those goals. My blood pressure went from 145 over 90 to a healthy 112 over 75 and my cholesterol went from 250 down to 194 and I lost about 50 lbs all in just a few short months. Now of course I didn't just do juicing, I made gradual changes such as eventually eliminating fast foods and sugary sodas, I also made a commitment to myself that if I had a urge for fast food I would just fill up on lean proteins and healthy juices until my cravings for bad foods went away and man did it work.

I was sure to reward myself for success, for every five pounds I lost I would cheat and have a couple slices of pizza or a burger but only at one meal. I don't cheat now as much as I use to because after 2 years of juicing and eating manly proteins, I really don't crave unhealthy foods as much. What I crave now more than anything is healthy foods. Sometimes I will even salivate when I see a banana sitting on the shelf because through repetition my body finally wants what it needs the most and that's proper nutrition. If I need a midnight snack I'll just prepare a healthy juice because that's mostly what I crave now.

If your body makes this adjustment and it should if you are disciplined, your cravings for bad foods should get less and less. It's almost like a drug addict weaning themselves off of heroin or something because I felt like I was addicted to carbs and greasy foods. The less often I had them the less my body craved them. See if you do a little work and strategizing you can lose weight pretty easy and one of the best strategies in the weight loss game is juicing, at least for me it was. I have never felt better and now I have more ENERGY than I've ever had.

These EASY DELICIOUS JUICING RECEPIES have helped me lower my blood pressure, bad cholesterol, improve energy, improve my skin complexion and I'm leaner and more fit than I have been in a very long time and you can do the same. It's time to take action for yourself and most importantly for your loved ones so you can stick around for them as long as possible and it all starts with what you put in your mouth. I know you will enjoy these recipes and have fun making them, I know I did.

2. Preparation for all recipes

Get yourself a really good blender. I like to use the Ninja because it blends my food up really nice. You may need to cut fruit and veggies in halves or quarters, it's probably wise to pre-package all your cut up fruit, put them in individual zip lock bags and store them in the freezer. This will help save you lots of time and hassle instead of having to do this every day, plus cutting up your fruit into smaller pieces will keep the food from jamming up the blender. For the most part the Ninja will blend up lots of whole fruits and veggies; it also has no problem blending up ice! I like to add between a ¼ to a 1/2 cup of ice to each juice because this makes a refreshing smoothie. If your juice ends up being too bitter try adding some bananas, this helps reduce the bitterness nicely!

3. Simplicity

The Simplicity recipe is a quick and easy juice I prepare for them mornings when I wake up late and have to be to work.

- — 2 carrots
- — 1 apple
- — 1/2 cucumber

Health benefits:

Skin benefit: Carrots contain vitamin A and other antioxidants, which helps prevent wrinkling, skin dryness, skin blemishes and uneven skin tone.

4. Fruit & Veggie Galore

I use this recipe when I want to make sure I got all the nutrients I need for the day.

- 2 apples
- 2 oranges, peeled
- 2-4 stalks of celery
- 1/2 cup of parsley
- 1 cucumber
- 1 lemon, unpeeled
- 1 small piece of ginger

Health Benefits:

Celery can help you lose weight because it makes you feel full without consuming many calories. Celery will also help you get your fluid needs as it is comprised of over 90% water. Having enough water in your body helps your workouts last longer. When you are properly hydrated it takes longer for muscle fatigue to set in.

5. Parsley Parley

- — 3 carrots
- — 1 large beet
- — 2-4 stalks of celery
- — A handful of parsley
- — 1 lemon, unpeeled
- — 1-2 cloves garlic

Health Benefit: Parsley's powerful oils can be an excellent health benefit because it is loaded with helpful antioxidants that help prevent cell damage which is a key in fighting cancer.

6. Kale Transformer

- 4-7 leaves kale
- 2 cups of spinach
- 1-2 apples
- 1 cup of grapes
- 1 small piece of ginger

Health Benefit:

Kale is full of powerful antioxidants. It is one of the most nutritious foods out there on the market today. One cup contains about 10% of the RDA of fiber, 9% of calcium and 8% of potassium. Kale has powerful anti-cancer properties as well because it blocks cancer cell growth, and increases DNA repair. It also has anti-inflammatory, cholesterol-lowering, and protective heart and respiratory qualities.

7. Granny Smith's Favorite

- 3 medium granny smith apples
- 4 stalks of celery
- 1/2 cup of Kale
- 1 lemon
- 3 cups of spinach

Health Benefit:

Apples are not only delicious and one of my favorite fruits to eat but they are extremely healthy for you. Studies have shown that apples may prevent bone loss; **Alzheimer's, help with asthma, lower cholesterol and may even prevent lung cancer.**

8. Spinach Delight

- — 3 cups of spinach
- — 1/2 cup of strawberries
- — 1 green apple
- — A small piece of ginger
- — 1/2 cup of blueberries
- — 1 cucumber

Health Benefits:

One cup of spinach has almost 20% of the RDA of dietary fiber, which helps in digestion, prevents constipation, maintains low blood sugar, and curbs overeating. Studies have also shown that the consumption of spinach may also reduce the risk of prostate cancer. I try to put spinach in all my juices because is has so many great health benefits.

9. Sweet Beet

- 1 large beet
- 1 red apple
- ¼ cup of kale
- 2 cups fresh baby spinach
- 1/2 cup of strawberries
- Spoon full of peanut butter

Health Benefit:

This sweet treat is one of my all-time favorite not only because it's so delicious but because it's so great for my body. Beets are an awesome source of many vitamins and minerals but they also act as nature's Viagra. Yep, you heard it right! The ancient Romans used them medicinally as an aphrodisiac. Who said we need doctors prescribing us with all kinds of pills when nature can provide us with all the healing and medicines we need.

10. Bunnies Favorite

- 3 carrots
- 2-3 stalks of celery
- 1/2 cucumber
- 1 green apple
- 1/2 cup of strawberries
- Small piece of ginger

Health Benefit:

This Crunchy superfood has many health benefits which include being good for your eyes, helps prevent cancer and promotes healthy skin. Carrots are rich in beta-carotene, the high level of beta-carotene acts as a barrier to cell damage done to the body. It also helps slows down the aging of cells.

11. Fat Melt

- 1 ½ to 2 cups of baby spinach
- 1 cup of Arugula
- 2 medium Roma tomatoes
- 1 lemon
- 1 small chunk of ginger
- 1 handful of basil
- 1-2 cloves garlic

Health Benefit:

Arugula provides a great source of folate, vitamins A and C, and more than 100 percent of your daily vitamin K needs. Not only is it a great weight-loss food, arugula can also help reduce your risk of bone fracture.

12. Six Pack, No More Keg

- 1/2 avocado
- 1 green apple
- 1 cup spinach
- 1 handful parsley
- 1/2 cup of kale
- 1/2 cup blue berries

Health Benefit:

Studies have shown that consuming blueberries helps individuals maintain optimal health because they contain vital nutrients the body desperately needs especially since the diets of most Americans today consist of mostly processed foods. Blue berries help improve memory, boost the immune system, improve eye sight and **neutralize free radicals.** These tasty little treats are packed with *Anthocyanin* which is found in the dark blue color of the blueberries. This powerful antioxidant helps neutralize free radicals that can lead to cancer and other diseases.

13. Firm Butt

- 1 grapefruit
- 2 cups spinach
- 1 handful parsley
- 1/2 cup of strawberries
- 1 green apple
- 1/2 banana

Health Benefit:

There is nothing like a tall glass of cool refreshing grapefruit freshly made from the Ninja blender. This amazing fruit has excellent health benefits because it's rich in vitamin c, it helps lower cholesterol and as a powerful antioxidant, vitamin C protects our bodies against oxidative stress caused by free radical damage and the inflammation associated with asthma and arthritis. Grapefruit is fat free and also contains a high number of fat-burning enzymes. Studies have shown them to also alter insulin levels.

14. Good Bye Cellulite

- 1 cup almond milk
- 1/2 cup of oats
- 1 Green apple
- Pinch of cinnamon
- 1/2 cup Blueberries

Health Benefit:

Studies have shown that as little as ½ teaspoon of cinnamon a day can lower your bad cholesterol (LDL). Cinnamon may help treat Type 2 Diabetes by lowering blood sugar levels and increasing the amount of insulin production in the body. Just the scent of cinnamon boosts cognitive function and memory. Cinnamon creates a chemical reaction that when consumed; the body actually reacts chemically to digest the cinnamon. This reaction speeds up the metabolism in order to offset the extra heat that is occurring as a result of the cinnamon. When the metabolism speeds up, you are burning more calories and you will lose weight more quickly.

15. Man Snatcher

- 1 small avocado
- 3 cups spinach
- 10 white grapes
- 1 cup of kale
- 1/4 cup flaxseeds
- 1/2 lime
- 1 small piece of ginger

Health Benefit:

Flaxseeds contain omega-3 fatty acids which is great for lowering bad cholesterol. Flaxseeds are also a great source of fiber and work as a natural laxative. Flaxseeds also contain Lignans which may protect against estrogen-dependent cancers such as breast cancer.

16. Curves in All the Right Places

- — 1 avocado
- — 1 handful of mint
- — 1 cup spinach
- — 1 cup parsley
- — 1/2 cup of strawberries

Health Benefit:

Avocados are high in beta-sitosterol, a compound that has been shown to lower cholesterol levels. I love to add avocados to most of my juices because they are a great source of protein which is great for muscle recovery after an intense workout.

17. Baby Got Back

- — 1 cup almond milk
- — 1 Cup of Romaine Lettuce
- — 1/2 cup frozen blueberries
- — 1/2 cup frozen strawberries
- — Pinch of cinnamon
- — A scoop of your own favorite protein powder (chocolate)

Health Benefit:

I absolutely love almond milk because it has less cholesterol then regular milk and fewer calories. One cup of almond milk contains only 60 calories, as opposed to 146 calories in whole milk, 122 calories in 2 percent, 102 calories in 1 percent, and 86 calories in skim. It makes for a sweat treat that will help you lose or maintain your current weight.

18. Makes Your Tongue Slap Your Brains Out! (Spicy)

- — 1 tomato
- — 1 cup of fresh parsley
- — 1 Cup of kale
- — 1/2 habanero pepper without seeds
- — 1 cup of romaine lettuce
- — 1 lemon juice squeezed into blender
- — Pinch of cayenne pepper
- — 1–2 pinches of flax seeds

Health Benefit:

I like to make this juice when I want something a little on the spicy side, like my grandfather use to tell me when he made his spicy tomato sandwiches, "This tastes so good it will make your tongue slap your brains out" and this juice is sure to do the same. Tomatoes contain vitamins A and C, these vitamins act as an anti-oxidant, working to neutralize dangerous free radicals in the blood stream. Tomatoes also contain lycopene which is one of the most powerful ant-oxidants known to man-kind. Tomatoes can also help repair the damage that smoking does to your body. Tomatoes contain chromogenic acid and coumaric acid, which help to fight against some of the carcinogens brought about by cigarette smoke.

19. Urkels Metabolism

- 4-6 large leaves of kale with stem
- 1 cup of Green Peppers
- 1/2 handful parsley
- 1/2 cup of cantaloupe
- 1/2 cup of blueberries

Health Benefit:

Not only are green peppers delicious but they are low in calories! You only ingest about 45 calories in one cup. The capsaicin in bell peppers has multiple health benefits. Studies show that green peppers reduce 'bad' cholesterol, control diabetes and provide relief from pain and inflammation.

20. Daily Glow

- — 1 apple
- — 1 lemon
- — 4 celery stalks
- — 2 large carrots
- — 6-8 stems parsley
- — 6-8 stems fresh mint
- — 1/2 banana

Health Benefit:

Mint is great for people who have acne and is sometimes used in facial cleansers for its anti-inflammatory properties and cleansing abilities. Using mint leaves for skin controls oiliness as it contains Vitamin A. It rejuvenates and refreshes the skin making it bright and soft! Consuming mint will be your natural way of getting oil-free naturally glowing skin.

21. Brain Food

- 1 Whole Spinach Bunch (About 4 cups)
- 2 McIntosh apples
- 1/2 avocado
- 2 oranges
- 1/4 cup Brazil nuts

Health Benefit:

Spinach is packed with an abundance of vitamin K that can prevent the break-down of bones as well as provide nutrient rich protein that is essential for maintaining the strength and density of our bones.

The large quantity of vitamin K in spinach contributes greatly to a healthy nervous system and brain function by providing essential nutrients that keep nerves in the brain healthy and functioning properly.

22. Love Handle Eliminator

- 4-6 cups of baby spinach
- 1 lemon, unpeeled
- 2 apples
- 1/2 cucumber
- 6 leaves of Romaine
- 1/2 Cup of chia seeds
- Optional: 2-3 garlic cloves

Health Benefit:

There are many health benefits in this juice to mention but probably the most surprising to me where the health benefits of romaine lettuce. I used to think that lettuce had no nutrients in it because I always heard about it being comprised of mostly water but after doing some research I found that nothing could be farther from the truth.

Romaine lettuce is the perfect weight loss food because it is comprised of almost 20 percent protein and it contains large quantities of cellulose and fiber which help fill you up without consuming a lot of calories. Because romaine lettuce has these things it is absolutely awesome when it comes to helping your digestion system. A healthy digestion system is extremely important in helping you maintain weight and remain or get to optimal health since experts suggest that the majority of diseases come from a poor digestion poor digestion system. Rule of thumb, anything vegetable that is green is most likely good for you since these things contain massive amounts of nutrients and healing benefits.

40 Delicious Nutribullet & Ninja Recipes!!!NEW!!

I just bought the Nutribullet a few months back because I wanted to see how it worked compared to the Ninja and I must say I like it indeed. Even though I am a big fan of the Ninja I tend to lean more towards the Nutribullet for the single serving juices and smoothies versus the Ninja. I like to use the Ninja for the big juicing's for several guests, but they both have awesome blending capabilities and are very easy to clean.

Kale & Berry Smoothie Blast

Ingredients

- ½ bananas
- 4 whole strawberries
- 1 handful of kale
- 1 TB honey
- 3 ice cubes
- Sweetened almond milk to the fill line

Health Benefits

The antioxidants and anti-inflammatory properties of kale have made health nuts go crazy over this fantastic leafy superfood; however, kale can be quite bitter and "grassy" in taste. This sweet creamy treat will help you easily consume kale without the bitter taste and it's great for selling your kids on a sweet and tasty treat while at the same time giving those many of their daily needed nutrients.

Green Spinach and Lettuce Smoothie Delight

Makes 2 glasses

Ingredients

- 4 cups chopped romaine lettuce
- 2 cups chopped spinach leaves (about half of a large bunch)
- ½ cup sliced celery
- ½ cup diced apples
- ¼ cup diced pear
- ½ cup sliced banana
- ½ tablespoon fresh lemon juice
- 1 cup of water

Instructions

Wash all vegetables and fruits thoroughly before handling them.

Put romaine lettuce, spinach and water together in a blender on the low setting.

Speed until mixture becomes smooth.

Add celery, apple and pear. Blend mixture at high speed.

Add the banana and lemon juice and puree until well blended.

Pour into glasses and serve fresh.

Variation

Add ½ cup each of parsley and cilantro for an even greener smoothie. Using the stems is okay; chop them so they do not ruin your blender or smoothie maker.

Add an inch of ginger to recipe for an extra sing.

Smoothie info:

This smoothie is designed to help you ingest more greens there for it will assist your body in absorbing more vitamins and minerals plus with all the added fiber it will help keep you full longer.

Sione Michelson

Green Energizer

Makes 1 glass

Ingredients

- 1 cup fresh spinach
- 1 cup fresh collard greens
- 3 medium sized oranges 3 cups pineapple chunks

Instructions

Squeeze out the juice from the oranges.

Use this fresh juice as liquid base for blending the spinach and collard greens together. Blend at slow speed until smooth.

Add the pineapples to the orange and greens mixture and blend at high speed until well mixed.

Pour and serve

Variation

You can add 6 ice cubes into the mix and blend until smooth.

Smoothie Info

This smoothie is packed with essential vitamins, minerals and proteins that is sure to give you an energy boost. Your body will thank you every time you consume this drink and each time you do you get closer to optimal health.

Papaya Oh My!

Makes 1 glass

- 3 cups spinach leaves
- 2 cups cubed ripe papaya
- 1 cup cubed pear
- 2 tablespoons blue berries
- 8 fresh leaves of mint
- 1 cup of filtered water

Instructions

Pour water into blender. Add papaya first, followed by the pear, berries and mint leaves. Add the spinach last.

Blend on high speed for about 30 seconds or until the smoothie turns into an even and creamy consistency.

Serve Fresh

Variation

You can replace the papaya with a whole banana which makes for a delicious sweet and creamy smoothie.

Smoothie Info

This smoothie recipe has plenty of protein, folate, magnesium and potassium. It's also high in vitamins A, B1, B6, C and K which is excellent for the skin and eyes.

Sione Michelson

Pina Colada Smoothie Delight

Ingredients

- 1 cup chopped spinach
- 4 cups fresh ripe pineapple chunks
- ½ cup shredded coconut meat
- 4 tablespoons dried pitted dates
- 2 cups unsweetened coconut water
- 2 cups unsweetened coconut water
- 2 cups ice cubes

Instructions

Put all ingredients in a blender. Remember to put the liquid first and the greens last. Add ingredients in between.

Blend on high speed until a creamy and smooth puree is achieved.

Pour into glasses and serve.

Variation

For a creamier taste you can even add 3 tablespoons of raw cashew nuts to this recipe.

Smoothie Info

Spinach is said to be one of the most powerful antioxidants known to humans. This wonderful green is packed with nutrients that prevent horrible diseases like dementia because it has folate, vitamin E, and vitamin K.

Kiwi Health Blast

Makes 1 glass

Ingredients

- 1 cup chopped spinach leaves
- 1 cup chopped kale leaves
- 1 cup chopped Swiss chard leaves
- ½ cup sliced ripe bananas
- ½ kiwi fruit
- Juice of ½ lemons
- 1 cup distilled water
- 1 teaspoon bee pollen
- ½ teaspoon maca powder

Instructions

Wash all ingredients thoroughly.

Prepare as directed in the recipe.

Put all ingredients in a blender. Blend at high speed until smooth.

Pour into a glass and serve immediately

Replace water with same amount of unsweetened coconut water for extra alkaline in your green smoothie.

If kiwis aren't in season, substitute it with mango or papaya.

Minty Smoothie Blast

Makes 2 glasses

Ingredients

- 1 cup chopped kale leaves
- 10 pieces mint leaves
- 2 whole pitted dates
- 2 tablespoons raw cashew butter
- 1 ½ cups distilled water

Instructions

Put all ingredients in a blender. Blend on high speed until smooth.

Pour into glasses and serve immediately

Variation

Substitute pitted dates with 1 tablespoon of raw coconut nectar or raw agave nectar.

Smoothie Fact

Mint is not only good for freshening your breath but it also aids in digestion and helps to sooth nausea and headaches.

Avocado Lime Weight Loss Extravaganza

Ingredients

- 1 cup young spinach leaves
- ½ cup sliced cucumber
- ½ avocado fruit
- 2 whole limes
- Sweetener (honey, agave or stevia) to taste
- 6 pieces ice cubes

Instructions

Wash vegetables and fruits thoroughly.

Take out the leaves of the spinach and discard stems.

Without peeling, cut cucumber into half-inch slices.

Remove see of avocado. Using a spoon, scoop out flesh from the peeling.

Peel and quarter limes

In a blender, place cucumber, avocado, spinach and lime. Add ice cubes and desired amount of sweetener.

Blend all ingredients until smooth.

Pour into a glass and drink fresh.

Variation

Add ½ teaspoon cinnamon powder to add some kick to your smoothie.

If you find your smoothie too thick, add ½ cup of cold distilled water and blend again before serving.

Smoothie Info

Sione Michelson

Limes are especially good for women's health. The citrus gems contain calcium and folate, two nutrients that are vital for post-menopausal women and women of child bearing age. Limes are also anti-carcinogenic and can help prevent the formation of kidney stones. Limes may even lower cholesterol.

Kale Health Optimizer

Makes 1 glass

Ingredients

- 1 cup kale leaves
- 1 medium sized Granny Smith apple
- 1 medium sized avocado
- ¼ lemon fruit
- 1 tablespoon sliced ginger
- A pinch of salt
- ½ cup distilled water

Instructions

Rinse kale in running water. Tear leaves apart.

Without peeling, core and separate apples.

Cut avocado into halves, remove seed and scoop out flesh using a tablespoon.

Peel lemon and remove seeds.

Peel ginger and cut into thin slices.

Put all ingredients in a blender.

Blend on high speed until well mixed and smooth Pour into a small glass and enjoy

Variation

Use limes instead of lemon for a slightly different taste.

Instead of adding sweetener like honey agave nectar, you can make this smoothie taste sweeter by adding more apples.

Sione Michelson

Instead of avocado, you can also use equal part banana in this recipe.

Smoothie info

Kale is another great superfood that is sure to help change your life by changing your health. Kale is full of chlorophyll which helps purify the blood. It also helps boost your immune system and clear lung and intestinal congestion.

Watermelon Smoothie Delight

Ingredients

- 8 leaves of mint
- 8 leaves of sweet basil
- 8 leaves of coriander
- 2 cups watermelon chunks
- ½ small avocado fruit
- ½ cup cucumber slices
- Juice of ½ lime fruit
- ½ cup distilled water

Instructions

Remove seeds from watermelon before cutting into chunks. Scoop out flesh from the avocado fruit. Slice cucumbers into half-inch thickness.

Put all ingredients in a blender in this order: mint, basil, coriander, water, watermelon, avocado, cucumber, lime juice. Blend on high speed until smooth.

Pour into a tall glass and serve.

Variation

Add ½ teaspoon of fennel seeds and ½ cup oats for a more filling version of this smoothie.

Put smoothie inside the freezer to cool it down for a few minutes before serving.

Smoothie Info

The health benefits of cucumber and watermelon are plentiful. Watermelons are mostly water, about 90 percent but this amazing fruit is filled with nutrients such as b6 and c, lots of lycopene, antioxidants and amino acids. There is even a small amount of potassium.

The health benefits of cucumber includes antioxidants, helps skin with its plethora of vitamins and minerals such as magnesium, potassium and silicon. Cucumber also aids in weight loss and cuts down your chances of getting certain cancers.

Apple Detox Smoothie

Makes 2 Glasses

Ingredients

- 1 cup shredded romaine lettuce
- ½ cup broccoli heads
- 1 medium sized apple
- ½ orange
- ½ cup distilled water
- 1 cup ice cubes

Instructions

Rinse greens under running water.

Peel and core apple. Cut into 1 inch cubes.

Peel orange. Remove seeds and separate into segments

Put all ingredients in a blender. Blend on high speed until thoroughly combined.

Pour into a glass and serve.

Variation

Add 1 tablespoon of chopped parsley into the mix for added kick.

Smoothie Fact

You have made and excellent health choice not only by purchasing this eBook which is full of recipes that will surely assist you in getting to optimal health but this particular smoothie is full of fiber, minerals, vitamins and phytochemicals that will assist in getting rid of toxins in the body.

Fig and Ginger Twist Smoothie

Makes 1 glass

Ingredients

- 1 cup spinach
- 1 cup figs (about 4 medium sized fruits)
- ½ tablespoon chopped ginger
- 2 whole pitted dates (pre-soaked)
- ½ cup distilled water
- 1 cup ice cubes

Instructions

In a blender, add spinach and water. Blend until smooth.

Add all remaining ingredients and process until blended smooth.

Pour into a glass and enjoy.

Variation

Add a tablespoon of flaxseeds for adding some kick.

Smoothie Info

Figs are a good source of potassium and minerals that helps control blood pressure. Fig is also a sweet way to lose weight being that they are a good source of dietary fiber. Studies have shown that postmenopausal women have had a reduction in breast cancer risk for those consuming the most fruit fiber compared to those eating less fiber and the Fig is a great fruit filled with the fiber one needs throughout the day.

Banana Smoothie Delight

Makes 1 glass

Ingredients

- 1 cup chopped kale leaves
- 2 cups diced ripe bananas
- ½ cup distilled water
- ½ cup ice cubes

Instructions

Rinse kale in running water and clean thoroughly.

Peel bananas and cut into 1-inch slices

Put all ingredients in a blender and blend until smooth.

Pour into a glass and enjoy.

Variation

For a sweeter taste, add 1 piece of apple (cored and cut into wedges) into the recipe. This will infuse your smoothie with the toxin removal properties of apples.

Smoothie Info

Bananas are Americas' favorite fresh fruit. This wonderful food is high in potassium and pectin; they can also be a great way to get magnesium and vitamins C and B6. Bananas are high in antioxidants, which can provide protection from free radicals.

Sione Michelson

Mean Green Machine Smoothie

1 Glass

Ingredients

- 2 pieces apples
- ½ a banana
- ½ piece cucumber
- 1 cup water

Instructions

Peel, core and cut apples into 1-inch cubes.

Peel banana and cut into 1 inch slices.

Without peeling, cut cucumbers into 1-inch cubes.

Place all ingredients in a blender and blend until smooth.

Pour into a glass and serve right away!

Variation

To make a cold smoothie, use only ½ cup of water and add ½ cup of ice cubes. Blend well.

Smoothie Info

A study shows that drinking apple juice could keep Alzheimer's away and fight the effects of aging on the brain, people who eat fruits and other high-fiber foods also gain some amount of protection against Parkinson's. Apples could also reduce your risk of developing pancreatic cancer and other cancers. Keep eating those apples!

Chocolate Green Machine Smoothie

Makes 1 glass

Ingredients

- ½ cup chopped kale leaves
- 1 cup chopped romaine lettuce leaves
- ½ cup Swiss chard
- 1 cup sliced ripe bananas
- 1 teaspoon unsweetened cacao powder
- 1 tablespoon natural honey
- 1 cup unsweetened coconut water

Instructions

Rinse and prepare greens and fruits.

Peel bananas and cut into 1 inch slices.

Put all ingredients in a blender and process until smooth.

Pour into a glass and serve immediately.

Variation

Add juice of ½ lemons for extra zest.

Smoothie Info

Cacao beans are seeds of the Theobromine cacao tree. They have chemicals called flavonoids, a type of antioxidant compound that promotes general health and might even lower risk for several diseases.

Sione Michelson

Green Giant Smoothie

Makes 1 glass

Ingredients

- 1 cup chopped kale leaves
- ½ cup Brussels sprouts
- ½ cup spinach leaves
- ½ avocado
- 1 medium sized green apple
- ½ cup filtered water
- ½ cup ice cubes

Instructions

Wash and prepare the greens

Scoop out the avocado flesh. Discard the seed.

Without peeling, core the apple and cut into 1-inch cubes.

In a blender, mix kale, Brussels sprouts, spinach and filtered water until smooth.

Add avocado, apple and ice cubes. Blend until smooth.

Variation

Add 1 teaspoon chia seeds for an added crunch

Add ½ cup broccoli or clover sprouts for extra greens

Smoothie Info

Brussels sprouts are rich in many nutrients. They have a great source of vitamin C and vitamin K. They also have an excellent source of other nutrients including folate, manganese, vitamin B6 dietary fiber, choline, copper, vitamin B1 and many other health benefits.

Pineapple Twist

Makes 1 glass

Ingredients

- ½ cup of fresh pineapple chunks
- 2 tbsps. granulated sugar
- ¼ teaspoon iodized salt
- 1 cup filtered water

Instructions

Mix sugar and salt in a cup of water, stir until melted.

Put pineapple chunks in sugar and salt water and soak for 8 minutes

Pour pineapple and water in a juicer and run juicer on high speed for 30 seconds.

Pour juice into a glass and drink fresh.

Variation

For a thicker and cooler alternative, add ½ cup crushed ice to pineapple and water mixture before running the juicer.

Add 2-3 mint leaves to the recipe for extra flavor.

Health Benefit

This delicious juice is an awesome fat eliminator because pineapples aid in digestion and help get rid of inflammation in the body by ridding the stomach and intestines of fat. Pineapples are also an awesome source of vitamin C, which gives protection from the flu.

Sweet Guava

Makes 1 glass

Ingredients

- 1 whole medium ripe guava
- ½ cup cold distilled water
- 2 tablespoons honey

Instructions

Wash guava and cut into halves.

Remove seed core and cut into 2-inch pieces.

Process guava and cold water in a juicer.

Mix honey in guava juice. Drink immediately.

Instructions

Use natural, unprocessed honey for better health benefits. Add honey to taste.

Health Benefit

Guava is great for weight loss because it has very little calories and it's delicious and packed full of fiber.

Banana Health Blast

Makes 1 glass

Ingredients

- 8 whole strawberries
- 2 medium sized ripe bananas

Instructions

Take off leaves and stems from the strawberries

Peel bananas and cut into 2-inch slices.

Put everything into the juicer and enjoy!

Variation

Add crushed ice before running in the juicer, this will make for a deliciously cold treat.

Add 10 pieces of pitted dates into the recipe for extra punch in taste.

For a sweeter taste, add 1 piece apple (cored and cut into wedges) into the

Recipe. This will also infuse your juice with the toxin removal properties of apples.

Health Benefit

Strawberries are high in antioxidants, which slows the aging process by blocking free radicals from the body's system.

Bananas are high in resistant starch, a type of fiber found in carbohydrate-rich foods that enhances fat burning.

Pomegranate explosion

Makes 1 glass

Ingredients

- 1 cup lychee
- ½ whole pomegranates
- 1 teaspoon food-grade vanilla essence

Instructions

Remove skin and seeds from lychees.

Peel Pomegranate and slice into 1-inch cubes.

Process lychees pomegranate and vanilla essence in a blender until mixed well.

Pour into a glass and drink fresh.

Variation

Throw in some crushed ice before blending ingredients together to make a refreshing smoothie.

Health Benefits

Lychees are low in cholesterol, saturated fats and sodium but they are high in copper, potassium, Vitamin C and dietary fiber.

Pomegranate is considered by health experts as a super fruit when it comes to weight loss. It contains massive amounts of vitamins and minerals that help detoxify the entire body, making you more vibrant and energetic. This amazing fruit also helps cut down on heart disease by preventing the harmful cholesterol buildup in ones arteries. You will also attain healthier more glowing skin complexion that is sure to make the prettiest person you know jealous.

Mango Paradise

Makes 2 glasses

Ingredients

- ½ small watermelons
- 1 whole ripe mango
- 1 ½ cup fresh pineapple chunks

Instructions

Remove the green outer rind from the watermelon. Slice the watermelon into 2-inch chunks.

Peel the mango and cut away the inner seed from the flesh. Cut flesh into 2-inch slices.

Process mango, watermelon and pineapple together in a juicer.

Chill juice for half an hour, then serve over ice.

Variation

Add one cup of cold filtered water to the juice to thin its consistency. Adding water will yield to three glasses of juice.

Health benefits

Watermelon is cholesterol-free, high in water content, low in sodium and extremely rich in ant-cancer phytochemical lycopene. Watermelon's high water content will help muscles become hydrated which will intern help reduce muscle fatigue.

Muskmelon Heaven

Makes 1 glass

Ingredients

- 10 whole loquats
- 1 small wedge of muskmelon
- 2/3 cups fresh pineapple chunks
- 2 tablespoons honey
- ½ cup cold distilled water

Instructions

Wash loquat and remove skin. Cut into 1-inch pieces.

Remove outer rind and seeds from muskmelon. Cut into 2-inch slices.

Process loquat, muskmelon, pineapple and water in a juicer for 15 seconds.

Pour into a glass.

Add honey and stir until fully dissolved into the juice. Drink fresh.

Variation

Serve chilled or over crushed ice for a refreshing drink during those hot spring and summer days and nights!

Substitute pineapple and honey with one whole red apple and one whole lemon for a citrusy, less sweet taste.

Health Benefit

The combined superfoods of the fruits loquat and muskmelon makes this juice a potent mix for removing fat around the mid-section and reducing cellulite around your hip thighs and buttocks.

Muskmelon has a plethora of beta-carotene, sodium, magnesium, potassium and vitamins A, B and C. It has large sums of dietary fiber and has zero cholesterol. Muskmelon also has a sweet taste, which can make any boring diet more bearable.

Papaya Passion

Makes 1 glass

Ingredients

- 1 small papaya
- 1 whole red apple
- 5 whole pitted dates

Instructions

Wash skin and remove the seeds of the papaya. Cut into 2-inch slices.

Wash and core pineapples. Slice into wedges.

Put all ingredients in a juicer or blender until a smooth juice is made.

Drink chilled or over ice cubes.

Variation

Add a teaspoon of finely chopped mint leaves to juice before drinking to add a burst of color in your juice and to make it more refreshing.

Dilute the juice with ¼ cup lime juice instead of water to further enhance the taste of papaya.

Health Benefit

Papaya is packed full of vitamins A and C, calcium, iron, niacin, potassium, riboflavin and thiamin, it's also low in calories and full of energy sustaining compounds.

Muskmelon and Apple Delight

Makes 1 glass

Ingredients

- 1 small wedge muskmelon
- 1 whole red apple
- 1 whole lemon
- ½ cup ice cubes

Instructions

Skin muskmelon and remove the seeds. Cut into 2-inch slices.

Wash, peel and core apples. Cut into 1-inch slices.

Peel lemon and remove seeds. Cut into half-inch slices.

Process muskmelon, apple, lemon and ice cubes in a juicer until a smooth juice is made.

Serve and drink right away.

Variation

Add a dash of cinnamon or cayenne pepper to help give your metabolism a boost.

Health Benefit

The presence of muskmelon and lemon helps ease symptoms of high blood pressure and regulates sugar absorption.

Fruit-topic

Makes 1 glass

Ingredients

- 2 medium red apples
- 4 whole kiwis
- 2 medium oranges
- 1 medium pineapple

Instructions

Core apples and slice into wedges.

Peel the kiwis. Cut into one-inch thick slices

Remove the outer rind of the oranges but try to leave all the white skin since it has lots of nutrients.

Be sure to removes seeds since this has a potential for making you sick.

Peel core and cut pineapple into spears.

Remove the outer rind of the lemons and lime quarters.

Run all ingredients into juicer. Stir and shake before serving.

Variation

Add ¼ lemons fruit and another ¼ lime into the recipe to make your juice more tangy and citrusy. Remember that adding fresh lemons to your juice will help increase your chances for weight loss because of the citric acid in the lemons helps kick the body's metabolism into high gear.

Health Benefits

Apples are an excellent source of pectin which is an enzyme that removes toxins from the intestines.

Oranges are filled with Vitamin C which helps reduce your chances of catching a cold. Oranges also help relieve constipation and inhibits kidney ailments.

Kiwis are rich in antioxidants and strengthen the immune system. Kiwis contain more Vitamin C than oranges, as much potassium as bananas and high levels of appetite-suppressing fibers.

Grape & Cactus Delight

Makes 1 glass

Ingredients

- 1 cup seedless grapes
- ¼ cup cactus pear fruit juice
- 2 small wedges of muskmelon
- 2 whole medium ripe mangoes
- ½ cup ice cubes

Instructions

Wash grapes thoroughly.

Skin muskmelon and remove all the seeds. Cut into 2-inch slices

Peel mango and cut away the seed from the flesh. Cut flesh into 2 inch slices.

Put all ingredients, including cactus juice and ice cubes, in a juicer. Enjoy.

Variation

If you cannot find seedless grapes, don't worry. You can juice whole grapes with seeds intact for additional antioxidant properties derived from grape seeds.

Use 2 whole, skinned fresh cactus pear fruit in place of fruit juice indicated in this recipe to get more raw fiber from the fruit.

Health Benefits

Grapes have a plethora of health benefits aside from losing weight. They are also packed with Vitamin C, boost energy, improve vision and inhibit the growth of cancer cells.

Cactus pear fruit (also called prickly pear) is an excellent appetite suppressant because it is rich in dietary fiber that will make you feel full. The fruit also lowers blood pressure and improves the health of the vascular system.

Beet & Celery Delight

Makes 1 glass

Ingredients

- ½ cup of cubed beets or 1 small whole beet.
- 1 cup celery stalks (about 5 stalks), chopped.
- 1 cup of spinach leaves chopped.
- ¼ cup of coriander leaves (about 2 sprigs), chopped
- 1 teaspoon salt

Instructions

Rinse celery, spinach and coriander in running water. Chop

Wash beets and cut into wedges.

Process all ingredients in a juicer. Pour in a glass and drink fresh.

Variation

Add a squeeze of lemon in your juice for a tangy experience.

Health Benefit

Beets are an excellent source of nutrients and are powerful detoxifier of the bladder, kidney and liver.

Celery is high in fiber, low in cholesterol and low in protein- an excellent weight loss veggie!

Cucumber & Kale Explosion

Makes 1 glass

Ingredients

- 2 whole small cucumbers
- ½ cup kale
- ¼ cup spinach
- ¼ cup parsley
- ¼ cup Swiss chard
- ½ slice lemon

Instructions

Rinse Kale, spinach, parsley and Swiss chard under cold running water. Without removing small stems, chop each vegetable separately.

Wash cucumbers and slice into 1 inch chunks.

Remove rind and seeds from lemon. Slice thinly.

Run all ingredients through a juicer. Pour into a glass and serve fresh.

Variation

Add a natural sweetener like stevia if you want to improve the taste of this mean green health juice.

It is best to drink vegetable juices at room temperature to preserve nutrients that may dissolve at colder temperature. If you should want to have this juice cold, pour juice over ice cubes just before drinking. Do not chill.

Health Benefit

Kale contains more calcium than milk, more iron than beef and ten times more Vitamin C than spinach.

Sione Michelson

All green vegetables effectively clean the digestive tract and the blood. Green juices are especially effective at giving people more energy as it also cleanses your body.

Asparagus Delight

Makes 1 glass

Ingredients

- 1/3 cup asparagus in cold running water. Cut into 1-inch cubes.

Boil 2 cups water and add asparagus. Cook until it becomes tender. Do not cook until it's mushy or olive green in color. Remove asparagus from water and dry. Set aside.

Rinse coriander in cold running water. Chop coriander leaves

Wash onions. Chop into 1- inch cubes.

Put asparagus, coriander and onion in a juicer. Add 1 ½ cup distilled water and sugar. Process until a smooth juice is produced.

Pour into a glass and drink fresh.

Variation

Squeeze a few drops of lemon to counter the strong taste of coriander.

For an added kick, add 4 thin slices of ginger before juicing.

Health Benefit

Asparagus is an alkaline based vegetable which makes it ideal for burning fat. It is low in calories but high in protein, folic acid, beta-carotene and Vitamin C.

Coriander leaves contain a host of nutrients, fiber, carbohydrates, vitamin C and minerals such as calcium, iron, niacin, potassium, phosphorous, riboflavin, thiamin and oxalic acid. Coriander promotes digestion and cleanses and strengthens the stomach. It is also a good diuretic (promotes the production of urine), which helps rid the body of toxins.

Splendid Carrot Juice

Makes 1 glass

Ingredients

- 2 medium carrots
- 1 cup watercress (about 15 sprigs)
- ½ cup spinach leaves
- ¼ cup coriander leaves (about 3 sprigs)
- 2 whole tomatoes

Instructions

Add 1 teaspoon of ground black pepper and 1 teaspoon of rock salt before juicing for an added kick.

Health Benefit

Carrots are high in polyunsaturated fats or good cholesterol. Carrots are also rich in fiber, which helps speed up the body's metabolism and prevents it from storing energy as fat.

Watercress is great source potassium, which serves as a diuretic to draw excess fluid from the body. Because watercress has more Sulphur than almost any other vegetable, it is excellent in the blood purification, protein absorption, cell building and promoting healthy skin and hair.

When consumed raw, spinach is an excellent source of foliate, manganese and vitamins A and K. Spinach is high in fiber and low in fat, sodium cholesterol and protein.

Broccoli Special

Makes 1 glass

Ingredients

- 3 cups broccoli (about 2 stalks)
- ½ cup chopped green bell pepper (about ½ medium whole)
- 2 cups carrots (about 4 medium whole)

Instructions

Rinse broccoli in cold running water. Cut into 2-inch pieces.

Wash bell peppers, remove seeds and chop.

Wash carrots, remove tops and cut into 2-inch slices.

Juice the broccoli, bell pepper and carrots together. Serve right away.

Variation:

Carrots are the most versatile vegetable that can be used in making healthy Juices. You can combine them with almost any vegetable or fruit and it will still taste good. Try adding a small apple into this recipe to make a sweet concoction.

Health Benefits

Rich in folate, manganese and vitamins A and K, broccoli is an excellent vegetable for losing weight because it is high in fiber and very low in cholesterol. You can help yourself with almost an unlimited serving of raw broccoli and you will feel satisfied without having to gain hard-to-burn calories!

Unknown too many, bell peppers are actually a good source of lycopene, beta carotene, potassium and fiber. Bell pepper increases your metabolism, controls your appetite and suppresses your craving for sweets.

Carrots are an excellent source of beta carotene, calcium, iron, magnesium, potassium, riboflavin and vitamins A and C.

Cabbage and Beet Delight

Makes 1 glass

Ingredients

- 2 large leaves of cabbage
- 1 small beet
- ½ medium cucumbers
- 4 medium carrots

Instructions

Wash all ingredients thoroughly

Roll cabbage leaves tightly into balls

Peel beet and cut into cubes

Cut cucumber into cubes

Peel carrots and slice into chunks.

Process all ingredients in a juicer. Drink Fresh!

Variation

Use more cucumber if you want to increase the quantity of your juice. Adding water will do the same trick, but using water-rich cucumber instead will add in more nutrients than water.

Juicing Tip:

When using cabbages in a recipe, you will extract more juice from the cabbage if you run it with hard produce like beets.

Health Benefits

Cabbages are extremely high in Vitamin K manganese. Those on high-fiber, low-fat, and low-sodium and low protein weight loss program will benefit most from incorporating cabbages into their diet.

Fruit and Veggie Extravaganza

Makes 1 glass

Ingredients

- 5 whole oranges
- ½ cup parsley

Instructions

Peel oranges and remove the seeds

Rinse parsley in running water, Leave for a few minutes to dry before chopping.

Put oranges and parsley through a juicer. Pour into a chilled glass and drink immediately.

Variation

For a fancy presentation, form two layers when pouring this juice into a glass by juicing the oranges and the parsley separately. Pour the orange juice first and then slowly pour parsley juice over it. The parsley juice will not mix with the orange juice and keep its place above it in your glass. You can just stir the juice before drinking if you do not enjoy the taste of pure parsley.

Juicing Tip

When Juicing oranges, remember to remove the outer rind but leave as much white skin intact as these are rich in nutrients.

Health Benefits

Herbs such as parsley figure well in a weight loss program because they aid in digesting and absorbing foo while providing a low-calorie diet.

Sione Michelson

Apple & Carrot Delight

Makes 1 glass

Ingredients

- 2 medium apples
- 3 medium carrots
- 4 Large stalks of celery

Instructions

Wash all Ingredients thoroughly

Core the apples but do not peel. Cut into segments.

Remove greens from the carrots. Slice into 1-inch cubes.

Cut celery into 2-inch sticks

Run all ingredients through a juicer. Pour into a glass and drink.

Variation

Add a dash of cinnamon to the juice and stir before serving for an added kick.

For added natural sweetness, put in one or more apple to your juice.

Health Benefits

This recipe is good for those who are still easing themselves into juicing and are not quite prepared for dark colored juices- you get all the benefits from the fresh and healthy ingredients without feeling "hardcore" about it.

Pear & Celery Delight

Makes 1 glass

Ingredients

- ½ cube pear slices (or 1 medium fruit)
- ½ cup diced celery (or 1 large stalk)
- 1-inch cube of ginger root

Instructions

Make sure all ingredients are thoroughly washed before preparing according to measurement indicated.

Run all ingredients through a blender. Pour over ice cubes in a glass and serve immediately.

Variation

For a creamier texture to this juice, process juice and ice cubes (about 5 pieces) in a blender.

Health Benefits

Pears act as a mild laxative while celery is a good natural diuretic. On top of this, ginger aids in proper digestion.

Banana & Apple Delight

Makes 1 glass

Ingredients

- 2/3 cup sliced bananas
- 2/3 cup sliced raw bitter melon
- 2/3 cup diced apples
- ½ cup distilled water

Instructions

Wash and then prepare or cut bananas, apples and bitter melon according to recipe specification.

Process all ingredients in the juicer. Pour into a glass and serve immediately.

Variation

Try adding a teaspoon of vinegar to the recipe to prevent color darkening of banana and apple due to oxidation.

If you still find the juice to be bitter despite the apple in the recipe, add a tablespoon or two of the natural honey to sweeten it more.

Health Benefits

Bitter melon aids in digestion and detoxification. It also helps regulate energy and fat storage.

Mango & Peach Surprise

Makes 1 glass

Ingredients

- ¼ cup mangoes
- 1 medium ripe banana
- ¼ cup peaches
- ¼ cup spinach
- ¼ cup distilled water

Instructions

Peel mangoes and separate the flesh from the seed. Cut flesh into 2-inch cubes

Peel bananas. Cut into 2-inch slices.

Cut peaches in half. Scoop out the flesh.

Rinse spinach in cold running water. Chop

Process all ingredients, including the water, in a juicer or a blender.

Pour juice over crushed ice in a glass. Drink immediately.

Variation

Chop 3 fresh mint leaves and add in the juice for a more refreshing treat.

Juicing Tip

The base ingredient in this juice is banana. Try it with any fruit and vegetable combination-like strawberries, pineapples, kale, Swiss chard or lettuce.

If you want a creamier juice, try adding avocados or coconut.

Sione Michelson

This juice is best taken as your breakfast, so if you are constantly in a rush in the morning, you can prepare this juice in the evening and just put it in the refrigerator. Juices and smoothies will usually remain fresh for 24 hours.

Health Benefits

Aside from potassium, bananas are also rich in fiber, amino acids, manganese and Vitamin B6. It is an excellent fat burning food due to its high content of resistant starch, which helps rid the body of excess fats.

Orange & Beet Treat

Makes 1 glass

Ingredients

- 2 oranges
- 1 medium sized red beet
- 4 medium sized carrots
- 8 pieces mint leaves

Instructions

Wash all ingredients thoroughly, especially the beets.

Peel oranges and remove seeds, but leave as much white pith as possible to retain fiber.

Remove greens from the beets. You may or may not peel the beets before cutting into 1-inch cubes.

Process all ingredients in a juicer. Pour into a glass and serve.

Variation

Add 2 medium stalks of celery to the recipe to further enhance the taste of the beets.

Juicing Tip

When a recipe calls for juicing vegetables and fruits with their peel or skin intact (such as beets and carrots), it is best to use organic produce since they are grown without the use of chemical fertilizers or pesticides.

Health Benefit

This juice is a powerful antioxidant. Although best to take in moderation, beets are good for weight loss because they are low in fat, fight water retention and help your body flush out toxins.

Sione Michelson

Pineapple, Carrot, & Lime Delight

Makes 1 glass

Ingredients

- 1 cup pineapple chunks
- 1 cup chopped carrots
- 1 tablespoon lime juice
- ½ small red or green chili
- 4-5 ice cubes

Instructions

Make sure all produce were washed thoroughly before chopping or juicing.

Prepare pineapples and carrots according to cut and measurement required by the recipe.

Slice the chili in half and remove seeds and stem.

Juice the pineapple and carrot juice, lime juice chili and ice cubes in a blender. Consume immediately.

Variation

For a more pulpy juice, skip juicing the pineapple and carrots separately and process all ingredients at once using a blender.

Health Benefits

This is a Vitamin C packed juice that will help boost your immune system.

Adding chilies to your juice not only gives a surprising kick but also helps in accelerating your metabolism.

Kiwi, Pineapple & Broccoli Delight

Makes 1 glass

Ingredients

- 1 whole kiwi, peeled and sliced
- 2/3 cup pineapple chunks
- 1/3 cup cucumber slices
- 1/3 cup diced broccoli

Instructions

Carefully wash and prepare all ingredients according to the recipe.

Run everything through a juicer. Pour into a glass and serve.

Variation

Add 1/3 cup crushed ice to the juice and stir before serving for an awesomely refreshing drink.

Health Benefits

Pineapples are rich in enzymes that will help detoxify the body by flushing out mucus build-up

Lemon & Apple Delight

Makes 1 glass

Ingredients

- 1 green apple
- ½ lemon fruit
- 5 outer leaves of red leaf lettuce
- 1 cucumber

Instructions

Wash all ingredients thoroughly.

Core apple and slice into wedges.

Peel lemon and remove the seeds.

Shred red leaf lettuce into salad size servings.

Slice cucumber into 2-inch pieces.

Process all ingredients in a juicer or blender. Serve over crushed ice if you prefer your juice cold.

Variation

Add ½ small ginger (peeled and chopped) for an extra zing to this juice.

Juicing tip

Red leaf lettuce will make your juice deep green in color with a smoother taste compared to bitter alternatives such as kale, spinach and parsley.

When incorporating ginger in your juice, expect to feel a slight burn in your body-that's ginger rousing your blood circulation and jumpstarting your body's immune system!

Health Benefit

Red leaf lettuce is rich in calcium, folate, iron and vitamins A and K.

Using ginger in your juice will not only give a spicy and citrusy taste; it will also help boost your immune system by shielding your body from viral infections and inflammatory conditions such as arthritis. Ginger also stimulates sweating which is important in discharging toxins through the skin.

Cucumber & Apple Delight

Makes 1 glass

Ingredients

- 4 red apples
- 1 small cucumber
- 2 large carrots
- 2 celery stalks

Instructions

Wash all ingredients thoroughly. Pay particular attention to the carrots, which tend to bind dirt and soil in their skin.

Core the apples but do not remove the outer skin. Cut into wedges.

Without peeling, cut cucumber, carrots and celery into 3-inch strips.

Process all ingredients in a juicer. Best served over crushed ice.

Variation

Use a medium sized cucumber to increase the yield of this recipe.

Health Benefit

This delicious juice is ideal for flushing out toxins and unwanted fats from the body.

Apple & Kale Special

Makes 1 glass

Ingredients

- 1 medium red apple
- 3 large leaves of kale
- 2 large leaves of lettuce
- 3 stalks of celery
- ½ medium cucumbers

Instructions

Wash all ingredients thoroughly.

Core apple but do not peel.

Cut celery into 2-inch lengths

Roll kale and lettuce leaves into balls and run together with apple or celery through a juicer. Add the cucumber chunks to juice together with the previous four ingredients.

Pour into a glass and enjoy this delicious green juice.

Variation

Add a small piece of peeled ginger for extra zing to your juice.

Health Benefits

The combination of kale, lettuce, celery and apple makes this juice a great cleansing juice that will help rid your body of toxins and unhealthy fats.

Carrot & Apple Health Craze

Makes 1 glass

Ingredients

- 2 cups chopped carrots (about 4 medium wholes)
- 1 cup quartered apple (or 1 small whole)
- 2 cups spinach leaves
- 2 stalks of celery (10 inch long each)
- 4 parsley leaves

Instructions

Rinse all ingredients in running water.

Remove greens and chop the carrots into 1-inch chunks.

Without peeling, core and quarter the apple

Roll spinach leaves into small balls that would fit into the feeding chute of your juicer.

Juice a chunk of carrot with spinach and parsley leaves. This process will help extract more juice from greens.

Juice celery stalks and then the apples.

Pour into a drinking glass and serve.

Add one small cucumber to this recipe to increase the quantity of your juice per serving.

If strawberries are in season, add 5 strawberries to the recipe. Strawberries, which go well with spinach, will help enhance the flavor of this juice. Drinking the juice of carrot and parsley will help you trim your food cravings because these vegetables are appetite suppressants.

Grape, Apple & Red Cabbage Flavorific

Makes 1 glass

Ingredients

- 1 cup seedless grapes
- 1 1/3 cup chopped apples
- ¼ cup coarsely chopped red cabbage
- 3 large stalks of celery
- 1 thumb of ginger
- 1 tablespoon balsamic vinegar

Instruction

Wash all ingredients thoroughly

Core and chop apples into 1 inch cubes. Chop red cabbage. Peel ginger and slice into strips.

Run all fruits and vegetables through a juicer. Pour into a glass.

Add balsamic vinegar and stir before drinking.

Variation

Add the juice of half a lemon fruit to recipe for a sweet citrusy taste to counteract the acidity of the balsamic vinegar.

Health Benefit

Don't let this purple colored juice fool you-it is packed with an excellent amount of vitamins and nutrients that is as healthy green as any power fruit and vegetable juice.

Just like your green cabbage, variety, red cabbage is rich in lactic acid, phytonutrients and vitamins A, C and E- but that's not all. Unlike its green sister, red cabbage derives its color from anthocyanin, an antioxidant that counteracts obesity-causing metabolic syndrome, insulin problems and hypertension. Anthocyanin also helps protect brain cells from Alzheimer's disease.

Apple & Beet-Sweet Potato Treat

Makes 1 glass

Ingredients

- 2 medium red apples
- 2 medium beets
- 1 cup sweet potatoes cubes (about one 5 inch long potato)
- 1 medium red bell pepper
- 1 large carrot.

Instructions

Wash all ingredients thoroughly.

Core apple and remove seeds. Cut into 1-inch cubes.

Cut beets into wedges.

Wash bell peppers, remove seeds and cut into half-inch strips lengthwise.

Remove greens and chop the carrot into 1-inch cubes.

Run all ingredients through a juicer. Pour into a glass. Stir before serving.

Variation

Add 1 medium sized orange to the recipe for a citrusy flavor to your juice. Remember to peel the orange and remove its seeds before juicing.

Health Benefits

Sweet potatoes are high in dietary fiber, high in water content, low in calories and low in sugar. It is thus an excellent addition to you weight loss diet.

24. In Closing

Again I want to thank you for checking out my book and I hope you enjoyed these delicious & healthy juice recipes. You now have one weapon in your arsenal (this e-book) that will surely help you towards the battle against fat and obesity.

I urge you to continue to add new weapons in your arsenal and if you have setbacks just keep going because all the hard work you put in will definitely be well worth it. I wish you a prosperous and healthy life, BE WELL SPIRITUALLY, PHYSICALLY AND EMOTIONALLY!

!!!!!!PLEASE don't forget to leave an awesome review if you liked my book; that would really mean the world to me!!!!!!

www.ingramcontent.com/pod-product-compliance
Lightning Source LLC
Chambersburg PA
CBHW071059290526
45795CB00004B/1573